FROM MANAGING TO CONQUERING ANGELMAN SYNDROME

Expert Guide To Overcoming Challenges and Triumphing Over Angelman Syndrome, One Step at a Time

DR. DASHIELL DANIEL

Disclaimer

This book, is intended to provide information and guidance on the subject matter and is not a substitute for professional medical advice, diagnosis, or treatment.

The author, is not a medical professional, and the content presented here is based on research, general knowledge, and expert guidance available at the time of writing.

The information in this book is provided with the understanding that the author and the publisher are not engaged in rendering medical, legal, or other professional services.

Any reliance on the information contained in this book is at the reader's own risk.

While every effort has been made to ensure the accuracy and completeness of the information presented, medical knowledge is constantly evolving, and new research may supersede the content in this book. The author and the publisher make no representations or warranties of any kind, express or implied, about the completeness, accuracy, reliability, suitability, or availability concerning the information, products, services, or related graphics contained in this book.

This book may contain references or mentions of individuals, products, websites, organizations, or other names for informational purposes only.

The author does not own or endorse any such entities mentioned in the book. Any resemblance to actual persons, living or dead, or actual events is purely coincidental.

Readers are encouraged to consult with qualified healthcare professionals for medical advice, diagnosis, and treatment tailored to their specific circumstances.

The author and the publisher disclaim any liability for any loss or risk, personal or otherwise, arising directly or indirectly from the use of the information presented in this book.

By reading this book, the reader acknowledges and agrees to the terms of this disclaimer.

The book "Angelman Syndrome" is an extensive and invaluable resource for researchers, medical experts, and anybody interested in learning more about this uncommon neurogenetic illness.

The first chapter of the book provides readers who are not familiar with the syndrome with a thorough understanding of its history and context. The target audience is specified, appealing to a wide readership that includes educators, caretakers, and medical professionals. The goal and scope are clearly stated, highlighting the need to spread knowledge about Angelman Syndrome.

An extensive definition, genetic origin, prevalence, and clinical features of Angelman Syndrome are provided in Chapter 1, which also explores the syndrome's basic elements. A more complex knowledge of the syndrome is made possible by the historical viewpoint, which provides insightful information on how our understanding of the illness has evolved. The examination of risk factors and causes, such as genetic abnormalities and parental imprinting, further deepens the reader's understanding of the illness.

Next, Chapter 2 delves deeply into the clinical aspects and diagnosis of Angelman Syndrome, clarifying behavioral traits, developmental milestones, and diagnostic standards. The use of differential diagnosis guarantees a thorough comprehension, assisting medical practitioners in precisely diagnosing and managing patients.

In Chapter 3, the genetic underpinnings and inheritance patterns are examined in detail, with particular attention paid to the intricacies of the UBE3A gene, the chromosome 15q11–13 area, and different inheritance patterns. For academics and geneticists, this part is an invaluable resource that promotes a deeper understanding of the molecular basis of Angelman Syndrome.

Important facets of the illness are covered in the following chapters, which include living with Angelman Syndrome (Chapter 5), treatment and management (Chapter 4), and research and future directions (Chapter 6).

These sections offer useful perspectives on treatment modalities, parental viewpoints, educational obstacles, and current research projects.

Finally, "Angelman Syndrome" serves as a vital resource that bridges the gap between scientific understanding and real-world application.

This book is an essential resource for those working in the disciplines of genetics, medicine, education, and caregiving because of the thorough examination of each chapter, which guarantees that readers obtain a comprehensive grasp of Angelman Syndrome.

Introduction

A particular collection of clinical symptoms, such as developmental delays, intellectual difficulties, speech problems, and a distinct behavioral phenotype defined by a cheerful mood and frequent laughter, are indicative of the rare neurogenetic illness known as Angelman Syndrome (AS). The original term for this complex disease originated in 1965 when Dr. Harry Angelman was the first to identify and describe it. The underlying genetic basis of Angelman Syndrome has been revealed through studies over the years, primarily involving defects on the maternal copy of chromosome 15q11-13. Even though AS is a very uncommon disorder, it has attracted a lot of interest because of its fascinating clinical symptoms and the difficulties it causes for those who have it and their families.

The Origins And Chronicles Of Angelman Syndrome

The origins of Angelman Syndrome can be found in the middle of the 20th century when Dr. Angelman first noted a set of kids that shared the same behavioral and developmental traits. Genetic research progressed over the next few decades, enabling scientists to pinpoint the precise genetic changes causing AS.

Understanding the molecular mechanisms behind the syndrome was made possible by the identification of imprinted genes on chromosome 15q11–13, namely the loss of function of the maternal allele of the UBE3A gene. Knowing the past development of AS helps to clarify its diagnostic path and emphasizes the teamwork that researchers, medical professionals, and families have put into deciphering the intricate nature of this neurodevelopmental illness.

Objective And Range Of The Book

This thorough investigation into Angelman Syndrome has several goals. First and foremost, it seeks to compile the body of information now available on AS by providing a comprehensive analysis of its clinical manifestation, diagnostic standards, and the most recent developments in genetic research.

This book aims to provide a useful resource for neurogenetics researchers, doctors, and genetic counselors by exploring the complexities of the illness. It also seeks to close the knowledge gap between science and practice by providing therapeutic interventions, instructional methodologies, and support networks for people with AS and their families.

This book's breadth goes beyond the conventional medical literature because it integrates multidisciplinary viewpoints from the social sciences, psychology, and education.

By doing this, it seeks to offer a comprehensive understanding of Angelman Syndrome, recognizing the various difficulties that people with AS encounter and the necessity of a cooperative, interdisciplinary approach to meet their particular requirements. The book also explores the moral issues that surround genetic counseling and testing, highlighting the significance of making well-informed decisions and providing compassionate treatment.

The Intended Audience

This book is designed to serve a wide range of readers, including families affected by Angelman Syndrome, researchers, educators, and medical professionals. This information will be extremely helpful to clinicians who specialize in neurology, genetics, pediatrics, and psychiatry as it will help them better comprehend the subtle clinical aspects of AS. The thorough examination of the genetic foundation of the illness and its effects on families will be beneficial to genetic counselors.

Educators and specialists in the field of special education will also gain useful knowledge for creating individualized lesson plans and interventions for students with Angelman Syndrome. These pages contain a multitude of resources that might help families navigate the difficulties of raising a kid with AS. This book aims to promote cooperation and knowledge exchange between several disciplines by reaching a wide readership, which will ultimately enhance results and quality of life for those with Angelman Syndrome.

To sum up, this book on Angelman Syndrome is an extensive and multidisciplinary resource that provides a thorough examination of the genetic foundation, clinical manifestations, historical background, and practical consequences of AS.

It aims to promote a cooperative and knowledgeable approach to the diagnosis, care, and support of people with Angelman Syndrome and their families by speaking to a varied audience.

CHAPTER ONE
A COMPREHENSIVE GLOBAL EXPLORATION
Synopsis And Definition

An uncommon neurodevelopmental illness called Angelman Syndrome (AS) is typified by a severe intellectual disability, speech impairment, developmental delay, and a distinct behavioral phenotype. Since Dr. Harry Angelman initially identified the illness in 1965, a great deal of progress has been made in comprehending the underlying causes. Angelman Syndrome is generally caused by defects on chromosome 15, more precisely in the 15q11–13 region.

This chromosomal area is essential for healthy brain growth and operation. People with AS frequently have distinguishing physical characteristics, such as a cheerful demeanor, a propensity for laughing, and an ataxic walk.

The intricacy of the illness is increased by the fact that affected individuals may experience varying degrees of symptom severity.

Genetic Foundation

Angelman Syndrome is primarily caused by mutations on chromosome 15. A deletion in the maternally inherited 15q11–13 locus causes the majority of cases (about 70–75%) and results in the loss of important genes. In other situations, people might have mutations in the UBE3A gene or inherit two copies of chromosome 15 from their father (a condition known as paternal uniparental disomy, or UPD). A protein that is essential to brain development and function is encoded by the UBE3A gene. The neurological symptoms of Angelman Syndrome are partly caused by the interruption of this gene's normal activity.

Incidence And Prevalence

Regarded as an uncommon condition, the estimated prevalence of Angelman Syndrome is 1 in 12,000 to 20,000 live births.

The incidence may differ among various demographic groups and geographical areas.

Both men and women are equally affected by the illness. It is important to remember, nevertheless, that given the variety of symptoms and the difficulty in detecting the genetic defects linked to AS, the prevalence may be misdiagnosed or underdiagnosed.

Clinical Features

Angelman Syndrome manifests clinically in a variety of ways, including both physical and behavioral traits. One of the main characteristics of AS patients is delayed or missing speech, which is one of many developmental abnormalities they show. Motor deficiencies such as ataxia, tremors, and a characteristic gait are additional prevalent symptoms. Most people with AS experience seizures regularly. Hyperactivity, difficulty communicating, and difficulty sleeping are some typical behavioral symptoms. Despite these difficulties, people with Angelman Syndrome frequently have a cheerful disposition, marked by a propensity for humor and an optimistic view of life. The distinct set of clinical characteristics demands a thorough and interdisciplinary approach to diagnosis and treatment.

Historical Angle

Dr. Harry Angelman initially recognized and documented the syndrome in three children in 1965, which marks the beginning of the syndrome's history. The illness was originally known as "happy puppet syndrome" because of the distinctive characteristics and behaviors of those who were affected, but in honor of its discoverer, Angelman's illness was eventually given the name. Our knowledge of the genesis and pathophysiology of the condition has greatly increased over the years because of developments in molecular genetics and neuroscience. The historical viewpoint emphasizes how crucial it is to keep up research efforts to fully understand the complexity of Angelman Syndrome.

Reasons And Danger Factors

It is essential to comprehend the causes and risk factors of Angelman Syndrome to make an accurate diagnosis and develop potential treatment plans. The main cause of AS is genetic alterations, and the most prevalent genetic anomaly is a deletion in the 15q11–13 area.

An important factor in AS is parental imprinting, a condition in which particular genes are expressed according to their parent of origin. The disease is caused by changes in the paternal silencing of the UBE3A gene in neurons, which is located inside the imprinted area. Additional reasons include mutations in the UBE3A gene itself and paternal uniparental disomy (UPD), a condition in which both copies of chromosome 15 are inherited from the father.

Mutations In The Genetics

Mostly, genetic abnormalities affecting the crucial 15q11-13 chromosomal region cause Angelman Syndrome. The majority of mutations found in AS patients are deletions in this area, which includes the UBE3A gene. These deletions could be inherited from a carrier parent or happen occasionally. The neurological abnormalities typical of AS are caused by the disruption of normal cellular processes caused by the lack of functional UBE3A protein production. Comprehending the particular genetic alterations implicated is essential for genetic counseling, prompt diagnosis, and possibly focused treatment methods.

Imprinting Of Parents

A basic biological mechanism known as parental imprinting is important for controlling gene expression according to the parent from whom it originated.

Parental imprinting of the UBE3A gene causes the expression of the maternal allele in neurons while the paternal allele is silenced in the case of Angelman Syndrome. The neurological problems seen in AS patients are partly caused by the loss of functional UBE3A protein as a result of this imprinting process disturbance. Understanding the complicated genetics behind Angelman Syndrome requires examining the delicate mechanisms of parental imprinting.

Mutations In Upd, Ube3a, And Deletion

The main genetic defects linked to Angelman Syndrome are mutations, uniparental disomy (UPD), and deletions in the UBE3A gene. Most of the cases are caused by deletions in the UBE3A gene's 15q11–13 region. When both copies of chromosome 15 are inherited from one parent—typically the father—uniparental disomy results, eliminating the maternal genetic contribution.

AS can also result from mutations in the UBE3A gene itself, which impairs the regular operation of the ubiquitin ligase this gene codes for. Because different people with Angelman Syndrome have different molecular pathways underlying the syndrome's etiology, these diverse genetic anomalies add to the syndrome's heterogeneity.

chromosomal 15 genetic anomalies are the underlying cause of the complicated neurodevelopmental condition known as Angelman

Syndrome, which manifests clinically in a variety of ways. Research is continuing to expand our understanding of this uncommon illness, from its historical diagnosis by Dr. Harry Angelman to the current understanding of its genetic foundation and clinical presentations. Investigating the complexities of genetic mutations, parental imprinting, and the various molecular pathways at play is crucial to improving the precision of diagnoses, providing genetic counseling, and creating focused therapy approaches for those with Angelman Syndrome.

CHAPTER TWO
DIAGNOSIS AND CLINICAL FEATURES

An uncommon neurodevelopmental illness called Angelman Syndrome (AS) is typified by a unique mix of clinical traits that affect many areas of a person's life. Examining the behavioral traits, developmental milestones, diagnostic standards, and differential diagnosis linked to Angelman illness is essential to comprehend the illness.

Developmental Checkpoints

Angelman Syndrome sufferers frequently show delays in reaching developmental milestones.

Fine motor skills may also be impacted, and motor skills like walking and crawling may be markedly delayed. Speech development is significantly compromised, and many people never learn to speak functionally. Furthermore, cognitive growth might not keep up, which would affect learning and problem-solving skills.

These delays underscore the difficulties that people with AS encounter in meeting developmental milestones and contribute to the distinct clinical appearance of Angelman Syndrome.

Behavioral Qualities

The behavioral features that distinguish those with Angelman illness from those without illness include a variety of unique attributes. Speech is either conspicuously absent or severely limited, which is a characteristic of communication difficulties. People could rely on nonverbal cues or communication gadgets as other means of communication. Sleep disruptions are prevalent, resulting in challenges in initiating and maintaining sleep, which ultimately affects the person's overall quality of life. People with AS frequently experience seizures, which makes daily living and health even more difficult for them.

Communication Difficulties

One of the most noticeable aspects of Angelman Syndrome is communication difficulties.

Most people with AS have minimal or non-existent functional speech, which makes it difficult for them to vocally communicate their needs, desires, or emotions. Even so, a lot of people with AS show a great desire to communicate and may come up with creative ways to do so, such as signs, gestures, or augmented communication gadgets. Their lack of speech has a substantial impact on their social and cognitive functioning, highlighting the need for specialized therapies and assistance.

Sleep Disturbances

People with Angelman Syndrome frequently experience sleep abnormalities, which presents extra difficulties for their general well-being.

These disruptions may show up as trouble falling asleep, waking up during the night, or waking up early in the morning.

Though not entirely understood, the underlying mechanisms causing sleep disruptions in AS are thought to be complex. Improving the quality of life for people with AS and helping their carers deal with the particular difficulties related to sleep requires addressing sleep-related concerns.

Convulsions

Since a sizable portion of those with Angelman Syndrome experience seizures, this is a serious medical problem. Seizures can come in a variety of forms and manifest at different phases of life. Comprehensive care for people with AS must include both understanding and treating seizures. Seizures can significantly affect behavior, cognitive abilities, and general quality of life.

Thus, to improve the management of seizures in people with Angelman Syndrome, routine monitoring, suitable medical therapies, and further study are crucial.

Diagnostic Standards

Clinical assessment, genetic testing, and meticulous analysis of the patient's developmental and behavioral traits are all used in the diagnosis of Angelman Syndrome. Clinical characteristics that commonly call for more research include developmental delays, speech impediments, and problems with balance or movement.

As the UBE3A gene is a characteristic of Angelman Syndrome, genetic testing—especially DNA methylation testing and chromosomal microarray analysis—is essential for detecting changes in the gene. To correctly diagnose and treat patients with AS, the diagnostic criteria highlight the significance of a multidisciplinary approach comprising clinical geneticists, neurologists, and other specialists.

Diagnostic Differentiation

A crucial step in the diagnosis process is separating Angelman Syndrome from other neurodevelopmental abnormalities. Angelman Syndrome and other conditions like Prader-Willi syndrome, Rett syndrome, and other genetic illnesses may have similar symptoms.

To confirm the existence of distinctive symptoms unique to AS and rule out other illnesses, differential diagnosis entails a detailed assessment of clinical and genetic criteria. To ensure the precise and prompt identification of Angelman Syndrome, healthcare professionals must collaborate and possess specific experience due to the intricacy of the diagnostic process.

Angelman Syndrome is a complicated neurodevelopmental condition with a unique combination of clinical symptoms. Comprehending the developmental milestones, behavioral traits, diagnostic standards, and differential diagnosis linked to AS is essential for precise diagnosis, all-encompassing care, and efficient handling of persons affected by this uncommon syndrome. The particular challenges presented by Angelman Syndrome require a multidisciplinary approach that integrates clinical knowledge, genetic testing, and continuous research efforts to improve the quality of life for afflicted persons and their families.

CHAPTER THREE
HERITABLE PATTERNS AND GENETIC BASIS

An uncommon neurogenetic condition known as Angelman Syndrome (AS) is typified by speech difficulties, intellectual problems, developmental delays, and an unusually upbeat attitude. Comprehending the genetic foundation of Angelman Syndrome is crucial to grasping the fundamental mechanisms and formulating efficacious therapy approaches. The primary genetic basis of AS is caused by anomalies in the 15q11–13 region of the chromosome.

Region Of Chromosome 15q11-13

Specifically, the 15q11-13 area on the long arm of chromosome 15 is the crucial region linked to Angelman Syndrome. Genomic imprinting, a mechanism that causes genes to express differently based on their parental origin, is present in this chromosomal region.

This region contains genes essential for neurodevelopment carried on the maternally inherited chromosome 15, and changes in this region are key to the presentation of Angelman Syndrome.

Gene UBE3A

The 15q11–13 region contains the UBE3A gene, which is a key component in Angelman Syndrome. The E3 ubiquitin ligase, which is essential for designating particular proteins for destruction, is encoded by this gene. Because it controls synaptic development and function, the UBE3A protein is especially significant in the brain. A prevalent feature of Angelman Syndrome is loss of function or dysregulation of UBE3A, which can be caused by a variety of genetic disorders in the 15q11–13 area.

Patterns Of Inheritance

Comprehending the inheritance patterns associated with Angelman Syndrome offers a valuable understanding of the various genetic pathways that contribute to the condition.

Erasure

About seventy percent of cases of Angelman Syndrome are caused by deletion of the 15q11–13 locus. This deletion might happen on the chromosome that is inherited by the mother, so removing important genes, such as UBE3A. The typical neurological symptoms of Angelman Syndrome patients are partly caused by the absence of functional UBE3A in the brain.

Disomy Uniparental (Upd)

When both chromosomes are inherited from a single parent, a condition known as unilateral disomy occurs, which prevents the other parent's genetic contribution. Paternal uniparental disomy (UPD) of chromosome 15 is a less common but important cause of Angelman Syndrome. In these individuals, the expression of Angelman Syndrome is caused by the absence of a functional UBE3A gene on the paternal chromosome, even though both copies of chromosome 15 are present.

Imprinting Errors

The epigenetic tagging of genes, usually based on their parental origin, is known as genomic imprinting. Imprinting errors may arise in Angelman Syndrome, resulting in the improper silencing or activation of several genes in the 15q11–13 region. The imbalance that is necessary for proper neurodevelopment is upset by this dysregulation, particularly in the expression of UBE3A, which adds to the clinical signs of Angelman Syndrome.

A Change In The Ube3a Gene

Although the most common cause of Angelman Syndrome is deletions in the 15q11–13 region, mutations that directly impact the UBE3A gene can also cause the condition. These mutations may compromise the UBE3A protein's ability to function normally, which could result in decreased ubiquitin ligase activity and abnormal protein buildup in the brain. The significance of UBE3A in neurodevelopment and the fine balance necessary for healthy synapse function are highlighted by these alterations.

the UBE3A gene is central to the complex genetic anomalies associated with Angelman Syndrome in the 15q11–13 region of chromosome 15.

The intricacy of this neurogenetic condition is highlighted by the variety of inheritance patterns, which include deletion, uniparental disomy, imprinting problems, and mutations in UBE3A.

To improve the quality of life and reduce symptoms for those who suffer from Angelman Syndrome, specific medicines that target the molecular pathways causing these genetic abnormalities must be developed.

CHAPTER FOUR
INTERVENTION AND SUPERVISION

A rare neurogenetic condition called Angelman Syndrome (AS) is typified by delays in development, intellectual disability, speech problems, and unusual behavioral traits.

Although there isn't a cure for Angelman Syndrome at the moment, there are several management and therapy strategies that try to enhance the lives of those who have the illness. The main ideas about the management and therapy of Angelman Syndrome are covered in detail in this section.

To treat the developmental impairments linked to Angelman Syndrome, early intervention is essential. Early identification and treatment of developmental difficulties is the aim of early intervention. Usually, a multidisciplinary strategy is used for this, involving the cooperation of medical doctors like pediatricians, therapists, and developmental specialists.

Early intervention programs may consist of educational initiatives catered to the child's individual requirements, focused therapy, and developmental tests. Angelman Syndrome sufferers may see improvements in their cognitive and motor abilities by treating developmental delays in their early phases.

For those with Angelman Syndrome, speech and language therapy is an essential part of a comprehensive care plan. One of the main symptoms of the syndrome is communication difficulties, which are typified by little or no speaking. Speech-language pathologists assist people with Angelman Syndrome in developing their communication abilities through a variety of methods, such as visual aids, sign language, and augmentative and alternative communication (AAC) equipment. The intention is to improve expressive and receptive communication skills so that people with Angelman Syndrome can interact with their surroundings and express their wants and needs more effectively.

For those with Angelman Syndrome, physical and occupational therapy are crucial parts of the treatment regimen. Common difficulties linked to the syndrome include poor motor coordination and problems with balance. Through specialized exercises and activities, physical therapists work to improve muscle strength, coordination, and gross motor abilities. Conversely, occupational therapists focus on activities of daily life, fine motor abilities, and sensory integration. The combined efforts of occupational and physical therapy help people with Angelman Syndrome become more independent and have better overall motor function.

Behavioral therapies are used to address the distinct behavioral traits that people with Angelman Syndrome exhibit. Typical behavioral traits include impulsivity, hyperactivity, and a propensity to project a cheerful attitude. The goals of behavioral treatments are to control troublesome behaviors, sharpen concentration and attention, and develop social skills. ABA, or applied behavior analysis, is a popular therapy strategy that emphasizes organized behavior modification techniques and positive reinforcement. People with Angelman Syndrome can have better social connections and a higher quality of life by treating behavioral issues.

Among those who have Angelman Syndrome, seizures and sleep issues are frequent comorbidities. To lessen the frequency and intensity of seizures, medications may be recommended for management and control. Medication and behavioral techniques can also be used to treat sleep disorders including insomnia or irregular sleep patterns. Healthcare professionals must regularly evaluate pharmaceutical regimens and make necessary adjustments based on the patient's response and changing needs.

For those with Angelman Syndrome, assistive technologies are essential for improving independence and communication. Speech-generating devices are among the augmentative and alternative communication (AAC) devices that can help people who are nonverbal or have limited speech express themselves. To encourage independence in daily tasks, other assistive technology, such as mobility aids and adapted computers, may be used. For those who have Angelman Syndrome, incorporating assistive technologies into daily life improves communication and increases autonomy.

A vital part of the holistic care strategy for people with Angelman Syndrome and their families is providing supportive and palliative care.

The goal of supportive care is to meet the emotional, social, and psychological needs of the person who is ill as well as the people who are caring for them. Palliative care is especially significant when considering Angelman Syndrome because it aims to enhance the quality of life for patients suffering from life-threatening illnesses. This entails treating all symptoms, providing pain relief, and offering emotional support while acknowledging that the illness is chronic and that it affects the affected people as well as their families.

a thorough and multidisciplinary strategy is necessary for the treatment and management of Angelman Syndrome to effectively meet the special problems posed by the condition.

The overall health and quality of life of people with Angelman Syndrome can be improved by early intervention, speech and language therapy, physical and occupational therapy, behavioral interventions, medications, assistive technologies, supportive care, and palliative care. Future studies and developments in treatment approaches could lead to even better results and assistance for impacted people and their families.

CHAPTER FIVE
LIVING WITH ANGELMAN SYNDROME

An uncommon neurogenetic condition known as Angelman Syndrome (AS) is typified by delayed development, intellectual disability, speech difficulty, and a unique behavioral pattern.

People who have Angelman Syndrome frequently have a cheerful disposition, laugh a lot and are fascinated by water. Angelman Syndrome presents special difficulties for affected individuals, families, and caregivers. To effectively manage the day-to-day responsibilities of offering care and assistance, one must possess resilience and a thorough comprehension of the syndrome's effects on all facets of life.

Parental And Caregiver Viewpoints

Raising a child with Angelman Syndrome is a rewarding and challenging process. In addition to juggling their child's special communication demands, parents frequently have to coordinate many therapies and navigate the complicated healthcare system. Seeing their child struggle with the restrictions placed on them by Angelman Syndrome can have a significant emotional impact. Parents' primary focus shifts to seeking medical solutions, educational materials, and therapies to improve their child's quality of life.

Parents and other family members who provide care are essential in fostering an atmosphere that is supportive of people with Angelman Syndrome. Because providing care can be physically and emotionally taxing, having a strong support network is essential. Working together with educators, therapists, and healthcare providers is essential to meeting the many needs of people with Angelman Syndrome. Building a sense of belonging and exchanging stories between caregivers makes the support system more knowledgeable and durable.

Opportunities And Challenges In Education

People with Angelman Syndrome face particular possibilities and obstacles in their educational journeys. The effects of the condition on communicative abilities and cognitive function call for individualized educational strategies.

To promote optimal development, early intervention programs, speech therapy, and augmentative communication aids become essential elements of an educational plan.

Despite being crucial, inclusive education comes with its own set of difficulties. Teachers need to be prepared to modify curricula and instructional strategies to meet the different learning styles of students with Angelman Syndrome. To create a welcoming and encouraging learning environment, special education specialists, general education teachers, and support staff must work together.

Inclusion And Social Integration

An essential component of the well-being of people with Angelman Syndrome is social integration.

The syndrome's distinct behavioral traits, such as a gregarious and welcoming demeanor, offer prospects for significant social contacts. However, social integration might be hampered by the communication difficulties linked to Angelman Syndrome, which can result in feelings of loneliness.

A multimodal strategy is needed to promote inclusion, and part of that strategy is educating communities about Angelman Syndrome. Informing classmates, educators, and community members about the features of the syndrome promotes acceptance and understanding. Through social skills training led by educators and therapists, people with Angelman Syndrome can learn how to handle social situations more skillfully.

Transition From Childhood To Adulthood

For those who have Angelman Syndrome and their families, graduating from high school and into adulthood marks a critical turning point in their lives. To meet changing needs and goals, people as they age require ongoing support and transition planning. The transition process revolves around independent living skills, work prospects, and vocational training.

A vital part of becoming ready for maturity is understanding the healthcare system, finances, and legal implications of guardianship.

To guarantee a seamless and effective transition, a cooperative strategy involving families, schools, medical professionals, and community support services is necessary. Promoting a feeling of purpose and fulfillment in adulthood requires acknowledging and utilizing the skills and abilities of people with Angelman Syndrome.

Advocacy And Assistance Groups

The panorama of advocacy and support around Angelman Syndrome is typified by the endeavors of groups committed to increasing public knowledge, advancing scientific inquiry, and furnishing impacted individuals and their families with necessary resources. These groups are essential in building a feeling of community, bringing families together, and promoting legislative reforms that will enhance the lives of those who suffer from Angelman Syndrome.

Raising money for studies that seek to comprehend the underlying genetic pathways of Angelman Syndrome and create viable treatment strategies is another aspect of advocacy work. Support groups work together with medical experts to share best practices for treatment, education, and intervention. Through enhancing the representation of people with Angelman Syndrome and their families, advocacy groups foster a more tolerant and encouraging community.

In conclusion, there is a wide range of experiences associated with having Angelman Syndrome, spanning from the time of diagnosis to maturity. The views of parents and caregivers emphasize the value of an all-encompassing support network, while educational opportunities and obstacles draw attention to the necessity of specialized interventions. The importance of promoting understanding within communities is emphasized by social integration and inclusion, and the transition to adulthood calls for meticulous preparation and teamwork. The voices of those impacted by Angelman Syndrome must be heard, and advocacy and support groups are essential in creating a more knowledgeable and understanding social structure.

CHAPTER SIX
RESEARCH AND FUTURE DIRECTIONS

A lot of study has been done on Angelman Syndrome (AS) to learn more about its underlying genetic pathways, clinical symptoms, and possible treatments. The main goals of current research projects are to discover new biomarkers for early diagnosis, clarify the molecular causes of the illness, and investigate cutting-edge therapy options.

Determining the function and development of the UBE3A gene and its protein product in the brain is one important line of research. Targeted therapy techniques can be developed based on ongoing efforts to identify the complex pathways implicated in AS pathophysiology.

New Interventions & Therapies

There have been notable developments in the search for effective treatments for Angelman Syndrome in recent years. From cutting-edge genetic and molecular therapies to conventional pharmaceutical treatments, emerging interventions cover a wide range of techniques. The goal of pharmacological therapies, such as altering neurotransmitter systems, is to lessen particular

AS symptoms. Furthermore, a potential area is gene therapy, which includes methods for increasing UBE3A expression or making up for its deficit. Utilizing CRISPR/Cas9 technology to fix genetic abnormalities causing AS is one of the novel techniques. The changing field of interventions is indicative of a paradigm change in favor of precision and personalized medicine.

Family Planning And Genetic Counseling

hereditary counseling is essential in helping families affected by or at risk for Angelman Syndrome because of the hereditary foundation of the condition. Genetic counsellors assist people in comprehending prenatal testing alternatives, recurrence concerns, and inheritance patterns. With the development of next-generation sequencing and other genetic testing technology, genetic counsellors are now able to provide families with more thorough and precise information. Family planning choices become more complex when taking into account the emotional challenges of parenting an AS kid, the possibility of recurrence, and possible carrier status. Making well-informed decisions and achieving better patient outcomes are two benefits of including genetic counseling in the multidisciplinary care of patients with AS.

Ethics In Research A Framework For Thought

As the field of research on Angelman Syndrome develops, ethical issues become more crucial in guaranteeing the ethical conduct of studies and the fair treatment of research participants.

A key element of ethical research procedures is the consideration of issues like informed consent, privacy protection, and the inclusion of various people in studies.

Utilizing cutting-edge technologies, like gene editing instruments, presents difficult moral conundrums because of the possible long-term repercussions and unexpected impacts.

It is a constant struggle to strike a balance between the search for scientific knowledge and the moral obligation to reduce harm and protect the autonomy of people with AS and their families.

To manage these challenges and promote a research environment based on honesty and respect for human dignity, ethical principles, and oversight procedures are crucial.

CONCLUSION

Angelman Syndrome is a complicated hereditary condition that affects afflicted people and their families greatly. Current research endeavors, driven by progress in genetic and molecular biology, are expanding our comprehension of the fundamental mechanisms driving the illness.

The development of innovative therapeutic approaches, like as gene-based therapies, has the potential to enhance the quality of life for people with AS.

To support families through well-informed family planning and decision-making, genetic counseling is essential. But as the discipline develops, ethical issues in research become more crucial to ensuring the just and responsible pursuit of knowledge.

To solve the complex issues surrounding Angelman Syndrome and to create a future in which all afflicted people have access to compassionate care and successful therapies, cooperation between researchers, medical professionals, and advocacy groups is crucial.

www.ingramcontent.com/pod-product-compliance
Lightning Source LLC
Chambersburg PA
CBHW071008260726
48661CB00007B/2856